HOLE IN MY SOUL

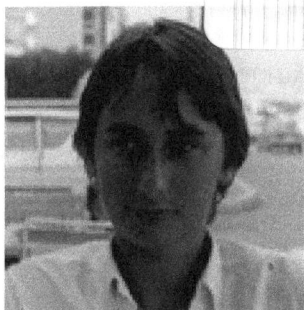

By Simon Russell

'One million people commit suicide every year'
The World Health Organization

Simon Russell

Published by
Chipmunkapublishing
PO Box 6872
Brentwood
Essex CM13 1ZT
United Kingdom

http://www.chipmunkapublishing.com

Edited by Heena Kausar

Soul Notes

Hole in my Soul is about my own unique, unusual and destructive journey. It is told in a collection of short stories called Soul Notes.

By the end of my journey I had lost everything of value:- My family, friends and emotional security. My career and financial well being. My house and home and my physical and mental health. A truly stunning descent from strength and order to weakness and chaos.

Most critically of all I had lost myself and I knew that without a clear understanding of my own identity I would not have the ability and confidence to regain any of what I had lost. This illness had destroyed my life and there was precious little that I could do about it.

When I have reflected on my life it is clear to me that I was almost certainly born with a hole in my soul. From a very early age I felt odd and troubled. It was not until I had completed my journey that the source of my pain was recognised. Too late because by then I had lost the battle against Manic Depression, culminating in the total separation of my body and soul. I had descended in madness several times and endured pepper gas, police detention, ECT treatment and several

3

sections leading to hospitalisation and the intake of powerful medication.

There were many people who journeyed with me, almost all of whom I cast aside in the desperate search for an illusive remedy to an undiagnosed illness. I simply could not fight the forces within me and as much as I loved my life and relationships I could not keep a grip on them. I was up against a power far greater than my own.

My journey has taught me about the importance of understanding and nurturing ourselves and our environment. Failure to do this fuels frustration, anger, violence and ill health. One day I hope that the really important issues of the here and now, poverty, pollution and disease are given the attention and resources they deserve.

The following collection of soul notes draw on my unique and varied experience of life to offer some observations that may be helpful in achieving this.

Simon Russell

HOLE IN MY SOUL

Life

Life is Love,
Love is life.
Hate is strife,
Cuts like a knife.
Life is Love,
Love is life.
Anger is strife,
Cuts like a knife.
Life is love,
Love is Life.
Dishonesty is strife,
Cuts like a knife.
Life is love,
Love is life.
Honour stops strife,
Love your life.

Simon Russell

HOLE IN MY SOUL

God Bless America

War torn world,
America can't be told.
Up their own arse,
MacDonald's a farce.
Prozac is the effect,
Cause they can't detect.
Naivety Rules,
Should go back to the mules;
Need for greed,
Generations of speed;
So obvious to see,
But absorbed by glee;
Vision they lack,
Too long in the sack;
Vice is the king,
It's all ding a ling;
They will fall from grace,
In front of their face;
The east will rule,
And the World will be cool;
Wish them well,
They just can't tell;
The world will improve,
Move by move.

Simon Russell

HOLE IN MY SOUL

Lost Sons

Boys have gone,
Not for long.
Time will cure ills,
Better than pills.
A lesson learnt,
Hearts can be burnt.
When things must change,
Time is the exchange.
Damage is done,
Mum, Dad and Sons,
Time to move away,
And let the clock play.
Boys need space,
And a slow pace;
Love will return,
With a slow burn;
When the pain gets bad,
Don't be Sad;
Visualise your dream,
Sun, Sea and Cream.

Simon Russell

HOLE IN MY SOUL

Italian Girl

A vision of beauty,
Mind body and soul.
Infected by a freak,
Invaded her whole.
Confidence dented,
But all invented.
Honest and sure,
Heart so pure,
Filled with passion,
Up with the fashion.
Looks great whatever,
Feels even better.
Dimples in her cheek,
Illusion of meek,
Eyes of green,
A lustrous sheen.
Fury and fire,
Never too far.
Fatal attraction,
A constant distraction.
Engaged in love,
A gift from above,
Completely at one,
Until it is done.
Saved a life,
Despite her own strife,
A giver for life,
A wonderful wife.

Simon Russell

HOLE IN MY SOUL

Green Gold

When he came second to Bush what could he do?
His opportunity missed, he didn't have a clue;
That he would have been better is in no doubt,
Cheated by the ballot box at the very last shout.
The messiahs of climate change caught his eye,
Suckered by statistics and the convenient lie.
It is a new gold rush with so few to gain;
Except for the shopkeepers where the benefits are plain.
Each new era is driven by a new fad;
In order for stockholders not to feel sad.
But the truth is that CO_2 is like a grain of sand;
A few blades of grass in an acre of land;
Doubled or trebled has such little effect;
So much so it is almost impossible to detect.
But profit can only be drawn by mass hysteria;
Selling gadgets and gizmos to the ever wearier.
It is also a governor of third world development;
Restrictions by the west their subtle new testament.
To make matters worse Blair has now joined the band;
The Al and Tony show will get a good hand.
But see through the mirror, see what is behind;
Don't be fooled by the rhetoric, don't be blind.
What is happening now is not born of human kind;
It is a cyclical event and a state of mind.
Not that we should indulge in waste and profligacy;

Simon Russell

Conservation must always be at the heart of our philosophy.

HOLE IN MY SOUL

Cold Fish

Post war stress,
Emotional distress.
77 years,
Plenty of tears.
Wanted to know,
Why love didn't flow?
44 years,
Plenty of tears.
Took to long a time,
To compose this rhyme.
Too many years,
Plenty of tears.
Inside's still warm,
Feelings swarm.
No more years,
No more Fears.

Simon Russell

HOLE IN MY SOUL

Death of a child

Where ever you are?
We know it's not far.
Your love abounds,
Beautiful sounds.
Mum is in pain,
Sees no gain.
An incredible loss,
We all give a toss.
Priests and Kings,
Have more important things.
Disease can be cured,
If money is lured.
We will do our best,
To prevent the rest.
Following your fate,
Before it's too late.
Not too long,
We'll sing the same song.
Where ever you are?
We know it's not far.

Simon Russell

HOLE IN MY SOUL

Hoarse Woman

Anger abounds at the slightest sounds;
Fury, rage and snivelling sounds.
As a young mare she didn't care;
Spoilt to death in a witch's lair.
Perfect ride, hid her feelings inside;
Father she loved, mother who lied.
Studs she attracted, but they all extracted;
When anger appeared from love it detracted.
For hoarse woman to prosper anger must go;
Soul searching, openness and truth must flow.

Simon Russell

HOLE IN MY SOUL

Reach Out

I want to reach out,
I want to touch the sky.
The harder I try,
The deeper the lie.
I want to reach out,
To leave a vapour trail,
But my life is stale,
Destined to fail.
I want to reach out,
Don't want to be plain,
But the pain won't refrain,
My soul has been slain.
I want to reach out,
I want the thrill,
But they tell me I'm ill,
Just take the pill.
I want to reach out,
At the speed of sound.
My spirit found,
Not flat on the ground.
I want to reach out,
I want to hear the bird song.
Please tell me what's wrong?
I am just dragged along.
I want to reach out,
How hard I yell.
Can anyone tell?
If I will go to hell.

Simon Russell

HOLE IN MY SOUL

Meatballs

It's a mystery to me,
Why we paid his fee.
Useless at best,
An unwanted guest.
Was his mind on the job?
More likely his knob.
When any old Nancy,
Would take his fancy!
The ingredients were great,
But as became his fate.
He was unable to mould,
A team fit for gold.
He swindled us all,
With his gentle call.
Leaders should have seen,
Beyond his sheen.
Our game paid the price,
Of FA and her slice.
Losing our shirts,
More interested in skirts.
As we return to the pitch,
Without Sven and his bitch.
Let's not be fooled again,
By a fraud and his feign.

Simon Russell

HOLE IN MY SOUL

Chameleon

A lion roars.
A lion fights.
A lion snores.
A lion bites.

A camel plods.
A camel chews.
A camel nods.
A camel phews.

Join them as one,
And you have a Camelion.

Simon Russell

HOLE IN MY SOUL

Psychospace

As I enter the world of Psychospace,
My brain and body no longer in place.
The final kick that hurls me out;
Happens so fast, no time to shout.
When I first arrive it's an amazing feeling.
Freedom, fulfilment and sexual healing.
King of the world, master of the universe;
Solutions for everything, however perverse.
No time for sleep, there are people to meet;
Got to spread the word and tell of my feat.
The answers are there to everyone's prayers;
Sent to earth down the ethereal stairs.
Tearing around fuelled by adrenaline and dope;
Preaching to the unwary, delivering false hope.
As the hours pass and the story is told;
Worry sets in, paranoia takes hold.
In this place there is no illusion;
My mind is not deranged, there is no confusion.
The power fades, the reality dawns;
My space is invaded by the devil's pawns.
Psychospace is a place where I feel;
Happy and strong and up in heel.
Everyone says 'you must not go again';
One of these trips you are bound to be slain.

But it's ok for them, they have not been
To Heaven and Hell and seen what I have seen.

Simon Russell

HOLE IN MY SOUL

Imagine the night

The sign says hospital but you are really not sure.
Unaware of an illness, no need for a cure.
The doors are locked but you can see inside;
Anxiety building like an incoming tide.
The door is released, you are welcomed in;
No uniform in sight, not sure of your sin.
Escorted to a room, another locked door;
Ragged and bedraggled, possessions on the floor.
The black sack is emptied, an inventory taken;
Increasingly nervous, frightened and shaken.
With all weapons of minor destruction removed,
You begin your internment until sanity is proved.
Long corridors stretch from the admin hub,
A T.V room with a patient battling a stub.
School like dining room, quiet between meals;
The soft furnished lounge where the spirit
congeals.
Off to your room, whitewashed and stark;
Signs of former patients have made their mark.
A radiator belts out interminable heat;
A plastic layer under the single bed sheet.
Washbasin and mirror, unbreakable of course;
The window designed to resist the greatest force.
An O.T. area to paint pointless pictures.
Doctors offices for your weekly fixtures.
Most important of all, it is why you are here.
The cocktail bar that dispenses its cheer.
Peace is broken with screams and cries;
Alarms are sounded, nurses rush like flies.

Simon Russell

This is not a place you would want to visit;
It corrodes your senses, things just don't fit.
You want to turn away, take rapid flight.
It's bad during the day, just imagine the night.

HOLE IN MY SOUL

Circle of Fear

If the haves have more, has a fundamental flaw;
Because the more the haves have, leaves less for
the poor.
In order to avoid hate, in a capitalist state;
The wealth must make sense, to the very last
pence.
Without a fair spread, only vice will get ahead;
Desperate to retain it's ill gotten gain.
When governors are attached, with whom are they
matched?
The people they serve or the evil they preserve.
If the system persists, only disharmony exists,
And all that is clear is the circle of fear.
Conflict is created, an illusion of hatred;
So that arms are depleted and orders repeated.
Peace will not prevail without a sting in the tail.
Whilst war boosts the coffers of the haves and
their officers,
It pervades the pores and opens the doors.
Because wealth is at the root of all those that
shoot.
Who do they protect? Only those they elect.
Who benefit in kind from the piper behind?
An enemy must be found, so the forces on the
ground,
Can be tested and tried to boost the presidential
pride.
The masses are scared, their freedom impaired.
As time after time they are subjected to this crime.

Simon Russell

HOLE IN MY SOUL

Paradise Discovered

As summer mounts the Everglades,
Visitors don their darker shades.
The ocean glisten green and blue,
The sunset has a reddish hue.
One end joins the Miami heat.
The other, the Caribbean beat.
An intermittent spine links both ends,
With bridges high above the bends.
The tranquil gulf opens out west.
The Atlantic east, a sterner test.
Islands, some less than a field wide.
Dotted down this great divide.
Pelicans glide the ocean top,
Dolphins play and never stop.
Manatees bask below the waves,
Rainbow fish in undersea caves.
Distant music from the Tiki bars,
Shoeless beings, open top cars.
A fisherman's dream, out on a boat
The big one missed or so he wrote
A wispy cloud in the deep blue sky
A welcome break, chance for a sigh
Paradise discovered in this place
Hemingway's hideaway puts a smile on your face

Simon Russell

HOLE IN MY SOUL

Searching

My heart beats harder as I await the call,
Will this be the one standing in the hall?
I check through the peephole, see who's outside;
Invariably beautiful, nothing to hide.
I open the door and welcome her in;
Immediately torn, feeling the sin.
I offer a drink, get her to talk;
I want to know what makes her walk.
A glimmer of light, a smile on the cheek;
Her heart shines through, mild and meek.
The thrill never stops, always a fix;
Soothing, sublime as our chemicals mix.
For her it's a job and normally shows;
Rarely involved until the action slows.
As the end finally comes and it is time to part,
Off with the skin and back to the start.
I wish her good luck and a fond farewell,
Another encounter for me to dwell.

Simon Russell

HOLE IN MY SOUL

Open Book

My best friend is an open book;
No malice involved, no stories to cook.
He makes friends where ever he goes;
His soul laid bare, his honesty flows.
My best friend is never too far
Always willing by train or car,
To visit me in my time of strife,
To soothe my soul and help my life.
My best friend is better than I could expect
Always consistent with his respect.
Never needing to check his speech
No sourness within, sweet as a peach.
My best friend will never forget
If he misses something he will always fret.
Scolding himself for being so lapse
Even with the little things, over zealous perhaps.
My best friend puts me at ease
Softly spoken, eager to please.
I know he is genuine, interested to learn.
What troubles my soul and makes me yearn?
My best friend has suffered too,
Advantage taken by an ignorant few.
He maintained decorum, turned his cheek;
Humble, compassionate, intelligently meek.
My best friend is to Africa drawn,
Too see for himself those less richly born.
He does all he can to help their plight
Acknowledging often the ridiculous fight.
My best friend has a heart of gold

Simon Russell

Discretion assured, integrity never sold.
Without doubt he's the person I trust
To read my words and spread my dust.

HOLE IN MY SOUL

Pharmacriminal

The power of the sixties revolution,
Created an inconvenient evolution.
Too many people with an enquiring mind,
Destabilising the future balance of mankind.
A regime where the leadership suppresses,
All but their own in their privileged addresses.
Supported by the giant corporations,
Controlling consumption and managing nations.
In order to stop this rising tide,
Some leading lights mysteriously died.
The plans and plots neatly concealed,
The people behind them never revealed.
The masses were affected too
To stop them being the next radical crew.
Pills and potions created in the laboratory
To ensure the populous did what was obligatory.
No danger to the money merry go round
Their sickening future safe and sound.
And we in innocence accepted our medication,
Completely unaware of this evil situation.
Has anyone the vision to resist this force,
To rise up and reject their course.
If such a being is really alive,
Please beat the goliath and let freedom survive.

Simon Russell

HOLE IN MY SOUL

The Here Frontier

How noble it is to travel up high,
How wondrous it is to conquer the sky,
How challenging it is to venture in space,
How satisfying it is to win the race.
How rewarding it is to go to Mars,
How enriching it is to discover new stars.

How much better it is to stay on earth,
How much better it is to deal with the dearth.
How much better it is to cure our disease,
How much better it is to quell the rising seas.
How much better it is to feed those that need,
How much better it is to terminate the greed.

How valuable it is to make this world better,
How much better it is, in this, to be the pace
setter?

Simon Russell

HOLE IN MY SOUL

Spiritual Father

Dear Father, where are you when I need you
most?
Are you for real or are you the Holy Ghost?

You were loved by the nation;
Your soul had formation;
Your words rang true
To the red, white and blue.
They ended your life in sixty three,
To stop you giving people their liberty.
In that car you had no chance,
They just didn't want peace to advance.

Imagine if you were still alive,
How much more love would survive?
Imagine if you had not had to die
If the bullet had passed you by!
Your words had too much meaning,
Especially for the conservative leaning.
Scared you would lead a revolt,
And release the people from their emotional vault.

Argentina was your original goal,
Freedom fighting was in your soul.
You would lend your heart, head and mind,
To any cause of a worthy kind.
But your actions angered the CIA,
In this evil machine you caused dismay.
So the hit was ordered on your life,

Simon Russell

An end to your mission of removing strife.

Dear Father, where are you when I need you most?
Are you for real or are you the Holy Ghost?

Your words and music a magical mix,
You smoked your weed and had your fix.
Songs of freedom, equality and love
Reggae rock inspired by God above.
Your music moved many to tears,
Released anxiety and eroded fears.
But it was too much for the powers that be
A shell in your body their guarantee.

Did your heart really give out?
Or was it mob rules you chose to flout?
They built their bank in the desert sun,
Protecting it with the barrel of a gun.
You of course were the star attraction;
Your act created endless satisfaction.
The greatest entertainer to be born;
Your heart and soul you would not pawn.

They silenced you in a prison cell,
But could not counter your magic spell.
You had right on your side and everyone knew,
But the world turned it's back and left you to stew.
After decades under Apartheid rule,
The masses rose up and broke through the wall.
And finally you were released from that terrible jail,

HOLE IN MY SOUL

Still strong at heart if a little frail.

Dear Father, where are you when I need you
most?
Are you for real or are you the Holy Ghost?

Simon Russell

HOLE IN MY SOUL

The Real World

The real world is where people give
Their time, their soul, they live to live.
Holding hands and lifting feet
Pushing chairs, eyes that meet.
The real world is where people share
Themselves, their hearts, they really care.
Reading minds, guessing thought
A helping hand, everlasting support.
The real world is where the clock runs slow
It's movement unimportant, no where to go.
Wandering, ambling, no hurry at all
Someone to catch you in case you fall.
The real world is where money doesn't matter
All that counts is tea and a natter.
What did we do before the world went green ($)
And dog eat dog took over the scene?
The real world is where our ancestor's belong
Oh to return and push back the throng.
Join together, we can lead a revolt
This is not progress, let's call a halt.

Simon Russell

HOLE IN MY SOUL

Die Nasty

When you entered the house the dye was cast,
Your body and soul nailed to their mast.
Your purity and innocence was much admired,
Your womb chosen for the future king to be sired.
You thought you loved the prince of charm;
A fairytale romance, blinded to his smarm;
A magnificent wedding, it was your day;
You won our hearts in every way.
The early years ran as planned;
He appeared to keep the vows of his wedding
band.
You frolicked and played, had some fun;
The seed was sewn and you had your son.
With the future monarchy now guaranteed;
You had served your purpose, fulfilled your need.
With this in place he returned to familiar ground;
To the one about whom, mummy originally
frowned.
His deceit unending, you had to despise;
No one interested in your heartfelt cries.
He was the future, eternally protected;
No sins he committed would ever be detected.
Desperately lonely, constantly annoyed;
You began your own search to fill the void.
When the divorce was eventually agreed;
You thought you had been finally freed.
From a life of misery and torment;
And the evil of the establishment.

But you fell in love with an age old foe;
And they saw much embarrassment and woe.
From that day forth your card was marked;
Their agents with you where ever you parked.
And finally they struck on enemy soil;
A mission ordered that no one could foil.
It was done so well it put blame in reverse;
A heathen act, completely perverse.
You maintained your honour to the end and
beyond;
With the people you forged an incredible bond.
We live in hope that the truth will be told;
Who knows yet, The House of Windsor may fold.
With those behind it locked in the tower;
Perhaps a more worthy dynasty will flower.

HOLE IN MY SOUL

School daze

My system was shocked; I was on my own;
Barely in my teens and left alone.
Deep in the country at the base of the downs;
Confronted by prefects wearing gowns.
Sitting on my trunk, head in my hands;
Stifling the tears from my lachrymal glands.
Off to the dorm, eight beds to a room;
In complete trauma, consumed with gloom.
After unpacking the rules are spelt out;
By a housemaster known to beat and shout.
The smell of pants and polish pervades;
There is no escape, depression invades.
Salvation comes when I get into my bed;
And no one can see the distress in my head.
Dawn comes too soon, the deathly bell rings;
The blissful sound of the night no longer sings.
Shouting and abusing seems part of the drill;
Everything I do is against my will.
Forced to be silent in the assembly hall;
My fear and unhappiness a solid wall.
The masters paraded on the school stage;
Making me feel like a cat in a cage.
Away to the classroom, time for learning;
But I am blinded by my constant yearning.
I look outside and see freedom yonder;
'Why am I here?' I constantly ponder.
I know I am not dumb but my results are poor;
Is it any wonder with my eyes on the door?

Simon Russell

The system didn't suit; it was not for me;
I needed something different that allowed me to
be free.

HOLE IN MY SOUL

Black Sheep

How does a sheep know it is black unless it is
told?
In the field with its flock there is no mirror to
behold.

Why do you inflict your thoughts on me?
Why can't you just let me be free?
I am not square; I must find the round holes.
No point in hauling me over the coals.
It's funny how you never wanted to know;
How I was built, how my thought patterns flow?
In your mind conformity reigns, 'just tow the line';
But that's not for me, I cannot simply say fine.
My construction is different despite your seeds;
I am sorry if your don't agree with my actions and
deeds.
Emotions were something never to mention;
After all it might require you to pay attention.
No one's to blame; it's trans-generational strain;
Cause of frustration and terminal disdain.
How could you know, when I did not know me at
all?
I should have been introduced to myself before
the fall.
How I so wish I was born in a different time?
When being different was not such a crime.
The chance has gone; it's too late to look within;
Another blackened sheep not sure of its sin.

Simon Russell

HOLE IN MY SOUL

Goodbye

Saying goodbye rips you apart;
Pinches your soul, squeezes your heart;
Tears on departure, hard to keep back;
So much to say before you crack;
Not sure if your paths will cross again?
Can't stand that thought, fight back the pain.
You try to cover all the lost ground.
Things never mentioned, secrets found.
Words are stuck, muscles taught.
Mentally stressed, emotions fraught;
You embrace each other one final time.
Your bodies talk as if in mime;
You mouth the words as you drift away;
You feel as heavy as you silently pray.

Simon Russell

HOLE IN MY SOUL

Super nurture

Sexy, seductive with a wholesome soul;
Nurturing her children a lifelong goal.
Exactingly honest, a heart so pure;
Sensitive, smart and timidly sure.
Fun and friendly, someone to trust;
A naughty streak, occasional lust.
Uniquely built, a perfect combination;
Feminine features, great determination.
Happy to take souls under her wing;
And let them be, what ever they bring.
Teaching and tutoring her second nature;
Always fair, a wonderful legislator.
She clearly inherited her father's gene;
Raunchy and racy but never obscene.
Emotionally strong, able to see each side;
Someone in whom her friends confide.
Her smile reassuring, deep from within;
Green and Blacks chocolate her only sin.
Because of her warmth you cannot say no;
She will always accommodate and go with the
flow.
It's amazing that she has this neat configuration;
With her own life devoid of maternal consideration.
She is a great role model for a nurturing
generation;
Ensuring her children are filled with elation.
Don't underestimate her guile and fortitude;
She will always defend her moral attitude.
Righting wrongs runs deep in her veins;

Simon Russell

A people champion, supporter of minority strains.
Beauty and brains through and through;
To her principles and feelings she will always
remain true.

HOLE IN MY SOUL

Cloud Cover

Let's not deny the third world its rightful evolution;
Because of greed and exaggerated CO_2 pollution.
Let's dig in deep and help them to develop;
Their poverty and disease we can envelop.
Let's not ignore their pain and hardship;
It's something we can beat in a generation's trip.
They deserve salvation; they are fellow human
beings;
Not inanimate objects like stock exchange
dealings.
Let's not sit back and just amass our wealth;
It's time for action and to apply some stealth.
Mountains of surplus, food, cash and aid;
That we need never worry about being repaid.
A new philosophy has got to take hold;
Global citizenship, radical and bold.
Myopia pervades the wealth in the west;
Let's open our eyes to this difficult test.
Let's stop inventing these excuses for inaction;
And give this mission some much needed traction.
Let's change our thinking and reach into our
pockets;
And switch expenditure from guns and rockets.
For all the third world's ills we have a cure;
What's holding us back is a greedy allure.
Let's give them life, let's allow them to be freed;
Let's teach them what we know and give them
what they need.

Simon Russell

HOLE IN MY SOUL

Palio

Dawn creeps up and lights the majesty of Il
Campo,
There is an eerie still before the storm of the Palio.
A magnificent theatre with tawny facades,
The perfect setting for this game of charades.
This race of pride is now ten centuries old,
The winning rider, brave and bold.

There are no saddles to keep them in the seat,
Getting round and staying on a marvellous feat.
The seventeen districts vying for first place,
Emotions' running high, this is not just a race.
Spectators flock and fill this natural stadium,
Waiting as if for gladiators in their coliseum.

The masses congregate in the centre of the ring,
An elegant few at restaurants in tiered seating.
As the day progresses and the tension mounts,
The riders know that it is only winning that counts.
The horses are taken to the chapel and blessed,
The shirts of the riders bearing their district crest.
At the starting rope the riders jockey for position,
False starts delay for some their lifelong ambition.
Finally they are off and race for the first turn,
The excitement now raging as the muscles burn.
Positions change as there are few rules,
Crashing and bumping, driving their mules.
It's over too quick and the winner is enthroned,
The King of Siena, for that day at least, the title is

loaned.

And after the finish the crowds flood on to the
track,
Fighting breaks out, tears can't be held back.
For all but the winner a gloom has descended,
Spirits forlorn and lives upended.
As dusk settles down and the fervour quells,
Tables and chairs and all round cooking smells.
The day leaves an imprint deep in your soul,
A timeless wonder, you feel more whole.

HOLE IN MY SOUL

Killing Spree

Images of death constantly on screen;
No holes barred, the gore always seen;
Glorification of violence, ratings must;
Bloody war games in the desert dust.
Whether on disc or a games console,
In invades the senses and withers the soul.
Locked inside, multi media at hand;
Broadcasted under an accepted brand.
Is it any wonder a young mind flips?
When repeatedly presented with unsavoury clips,
With the brain being such a complex place,
And the world moving at an ungodly pace.
Research is needed to see if there is a video link,
That takes the killer beyond the brink.
It may just be all a troubled soul needs,
To pull the trigger and commit these deeds.
Let's try and get inside the mind,
And see what connections we can find.
So that future generations can learn in peace,
And the killers won't need this tension release.

Simon Russell

HOLE IN MY SOUL

Lost

Where am I now, I'm totally lost;
Chilled to the bone, cold as frost.
I entered the maze some time ago;
Impenetrable walls, no directional flow.
In so deep, there is no way back;
No light in sight, just very dark black.
I am not at all sure how I ventured in;
Looking for something, perhaps new love to win.
I have been inside such a terribly long time;
My life before forgotten, so sublime.
No sense of the future without an exit route;
I pray for a gun and someone to shoot.
I often feel dizzy, totally out of sorts;
A ship in an ocean without any ports.
Where are the signs, recognition wiped clean?
No benchmarks around, nothing to glean;
Hopelessly, helplessly, haplessly estranged.
Heading nowhere, worryingly deranged;
Running out of energy, little fuel in the tank;
No one to blame, only myself to thank.
Hoping still for a miracle to occur,
That might save my soul and the inevitable defer.

Simon Russell

HOLE IN MY SOUL

Iron Maiden

Born to a grocer, feet on the ground;
No silver spoon, no silken sound;
Determination in bred at birth;
Able to resist criticism and mirth.
Principled and honest through and through;
A natural born leader, of which there are few;
Her policies I disputed but she was still one to admire;
Her steely resolve, that went to the wire.
She rid the nation of its hurtful shackles;
Never shying from the dangerous tackles;
No weakness exposed on her face;
Her guarantee not to fall from grace.
Always at ease at the negotiating table;
Winning minds, establishing her label;
The Russians and Americans, her genuine friends;
Brokering harmony, straightening the bends.
Her nations interest constantly at heart;
Selflessly toiling, assured and smart;
Restoring pride to this crestfallen place;
Rebuilding confidence with steel and grace.
When an adversary invaded her land;
She rallied the troops and conducted the band;
Repelling the forces that arrived at Stanley;
Re-raising her flag, proud, strong and manly.
Her termination was a very sad day;
Not fitting for a leader who succeeded in her way;
Amongst the greats she will always sit;

Simon Russell

At home with Gladstone, Churchill and Pitt.

HOLE IN MY SOUL

The Great Pretender

He will be remembered as the great teller of lies;
Darkness, deceit and warmongering cries.
He came to power on a tide of glory;
No opposition to counter his pious story.
The US model was his claim to fame;
Riddled with corruption, the corporate game.
How we were fooled by his evil stare?
And the constant chants of 'vote for Blair'.
He repaid his backers with honours galore;
High powered jobs, titles and more.
But his only interest was self preservation,
Remembered as the saviour of the nation,
And to prepare for his later luminary career;
Buying new friendships, year after year.
His lasting legacy, the war in Iraq,
With Bush the dog and Blair the bark.
This cosy relationship immoral and black,
Throughout the turmoil he dodged the flack.
The blood of many indelibly printed;
His soul won't suffer, his medal already minted.
David Kelly's death ordered to cover his sin;
He knew too much and 'NO 'votes could win.
His followers bizarrely aped his every word;
Like lambs to the slaughter, a characterless herd.
Its ironic his initials are the same as a foul
disease;
How many has he killed in his attempts to
appease?
Yes of course he is the great pretender;

Simon Russell

For the worst PM he is the best contender.

HOLE IN MY SOUL

Another case of the Blues

Social responsibility is a pile of crap,
Just another political rap.
Something for the minority majority to hear,
So that to the blues they may endear.
In reality there is no original thought,
And what has Cameron really brought.
A carbon copy of the nasty Blair,
In many ways a natural heir.
Without a pedigree at the grass roots,
Happier with the band that hunts and shoots.
Custom made by the media machine,
Beautiful coiffure, slick and lean.
Well briefed, confident and sure,
Of societies ills he promises a cure.
But his eyes give away the traitor inside,
And in no time, despite tricks he will have tried.
The true blue colours will be back on show,
As he screws the people and lies flow and flow.

Simon Russell

HOLE IN MY SOUL

Afterlife

It has always been life's great mystery,
With numerous theories throughout history.
The solution to this riddle is simple to me,
Because of my experiences it's easy to see.
When your life has passed you can only dream,
Stuck in the afterlife, no matter what you scream.
Your soul is locked in, there is no way out;
What ever your position, you have no clout.
As in life your dreams can be good or bad;
Exceptionally happy or terrifyingly sad.
This then is what they call Heaven and Hell;
And which you enter only you can tell.
All will be determined by your life on earth;
And what you have done since the day of your
birth.
Your afterlife destiny controlled by your own
deeds;
How you have behaved and sewn your seeds?
So live with a conscience and sew them well,
Nurture your life, create a positive shell.
It will serve you right in your afterlife,
Your permanent dream free from all strife.

Simon Russell

HOLE IN MY SOUL

Milky Way

No one understands a boy like a boy;
Tried by many as an innocent ploy.
Touching and feeling, initial exploration;
Nothing invasive, just mutual experimentation.
Gripping hand to a foreign member;
A fast heart beat to always remember.
Face to face feels a little rough;
Outside action is plenty enough.
Forbidden fruit is part of the thrill;
Keeping it quiet, laying still.
Eyes and ears waiting to catch;
This illicit lust on their patch.
What can be expected with boys together?
And no other outlet for their soul to tether.
Part of life's learning lessons,
Preparation for future adult sessions.
Which ever way you end up leaning;
It helps to give sex greater meaning.
To feel for yourself the Milky Way;
You to understand that it is more than a lay.
No need for regret or to feel you soiled;
You have had the experience of a spring uncoiled.

Simon Russell

HOLE IN MY SOUL

Ring Road

I started and finished in exactly the same place,
Around the ring road at double the pace;
Now back at the beginning with nowhere to go,
The end of the road and the end of the show.

No earlier memories before the crack to my head,
The scar a talking point in the life I've led;
But was the damage deeper than first thought,
Did it create the hole in which my life was caught?

I had some successes along the way,
Reasons for joy at work and play;
But continuity evaded me, difficult to sustain,
The twists and turns only causing pain.

The highest of highs, the birth of my boys,
Watching them grow and playing with their toys;
Determined not to be a part time dad,
But alone now without them and terribly sad.

All I wanted was a life by the sea,
My wife, my children, my work and me;
To hear the sound of gulls and waves,
My family and me not consumer slaves.

I experienced the rush of love in my veins,
Like a connection direct to the mains;
But my illness took over and I had to let go,
To preserve her own soul and let her life flow.

Simon Russell

There was a period of bliss in my mid to late
twenties,
When life seemed to pass with consummate ease;
But it wasn't enough; I had a hunger for more,
With my foot on the accelerator, I hit the floor.

Going so fast I lost sight of the road,
A breakdown inevitable, I could not be slowed;
Blinded by bright lights and the rush for success,
I ignored the warnings and drove to excess.

I was sent for repairs and wired to the mains,
I had lost control, let go of the reigns;
From that day forward life was never the same,
It was struggle after struggle as I lost the game.

I had my heroes, John Lennon and Che,
Elvis, Mandela, Bob Marley and JFK.
But they were rich in spirit and their souls
complete,
With their achievements I could hardly compete.

As I look in the mirror it seems a shameful waste,
A journey taken in too much haste;
Blighted by drugs, hubris and greed,
And so many things that I did not need.

At some point or another around the track,
Perhaps from birth, I was only able to see black;
It rendered me weak, far from whole;
For I lived my life with a hole in my soul.

HOLE IN MY SOUL

Jamaica Cake

The smell is arresting, it excites the senses;
Once experienced it will override any defences.
It crumbles beautifully in the fingers when warm;
Deep in the gut, feelings of anticipation swarm.
Rolled with tobacco into a neat spliff;
The heart beats faster waiting for the first whiff.
Drawing it down gives a wonderful smooth kick;
Inhaling the fumes brings it on easy and quick.
Reality fades, words escape but sense evades;
Lost in space, weightlessness pervades.
In a place of your own, no pain in sight;
Briefly at peace, troubles have taken flight.
Before too long realisation takes hold;
It's not a permanent state, expectations fold.
The pain returns, harsher with each time;
Terror takes hold and repays the crime.
It's really not worth the momentary trip;
Even if it gives you an upward blip.
The damage to the brain is evidence itself;
That this is a product to be left on the shelf.
The years that follow can be constant torture;
Whatever the substance, however pure;
Of course there is proper and positive spin,
But this is in an attempt for the addiction to win.
Once in your blood stream it's impossible to
refuse;
Stop before starting, there is really nothing to lose.

Simon Russell

HOLE IN MY SOUL

Magic Box

A means of communication, a method to control;
This vacuous box sucks in the soul.
Its invention great, its intention to entertain;
But it was quickly ambushed by those who inflict
pain.
Propaganda sprang forth to give a positive spin;
To protect those in power and hearts to win.
Images of war brought into everyone's room;
Propagating fantasy, much gloom and doom.
This served to instil fear against a common foe;
And secure their position with each terrifying blow.
Of its bias there is absolutely no doubt;
Little objectivity, governed by media clout.
Power and projection so closely entwined;
The interests of the people rarely defined.
Broadcasting suffering is a ratings success;
Enabling the barons to live life to excess.
But what of the minds of those who watch;
Not suspecting brain washing from their top notch.
Good God, we in the west are whiter than white;
We hold the moral high ground, never start the
fight.
The grand illusion maintained through the magic
box;
Delicately mind bending, sly as a fox.

Simon Russell

HOLE IN MY SOUL

The Burning Bush

A soul so black, burnt and charred;
A mind so twisted, heartless and hard;
A brain so empty, ignorant and dumb;
A heart so dry, emotionless and numb;
How on earth is our earth in his hands?
No intelligence, no knowledge of foreign lands;
A simpleton with hunger to make his mark;
No more dangerous combination, none so stark.
In cahoots with terrorists in the Arab states;
Lining his pockets from his wealthy mates.
His only determination to protect the oil;
Without a care of the damage to foreign soil.
He feigns his sorrow at the body bags;
Just pawns in his game, just metal tags.
His disquiet and discomfort easy to see;
Covered with bluster, bullshit and glee.
To a nation naïve and self absorbed;
His reign protected, his reputation not daubed.
But to the rest of the planet he is evil to the core;
Unless you profit from poverty and war;
Whoever is next they surely cannot be worse;
Than Bush the devil, immoral and perverse.

www.ingramcontent.com/pod-product-compliance
Lightning Source LLC
Chambersburg PA
CBHW031219270326
41931CB00006B/616